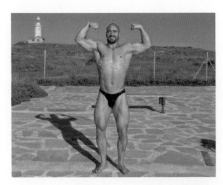

THE

HERCULES

FORMULA

12 Week Training Programme

UNLOCK YOUR POTENTIAL

A structured plan designed to maximise muscle size and increase strength

Max Glover

Contents

12 Week Hercules Power Building Training Programme

The programme will consist of 5- 6 training days per week.

All workouts MUST begin with a warm up of 7-10 minutes to prepare you, and every workout must end with a cool down and stretches.

For warm up follow this protocol:

RAISE body temperature by doing light cardio such a cycling, jogging or cross trainer. Gradually increase the intensity over at least 5 minutes.

ACTIVATE your muscles, focus particularly on activating your glutes and core, exercises like hip thrusts, side lying hip abduction and bulgarian split squats are ideal for this, 15 – 20 reps of each should suffice.

MOBILISE your joints – this will enable you to have a better and smoother range of motion while you are exercising. This can be achieved with exercises such a shoulder circles, hip rotations and bodyweight exercises.

POTENTIATE the muscles you are going to be using. Perform the exercises you are going to be doing several times prior to your work set, start off with a light weight and gradually increase it whilst focusing on your form.

If at any point during exercise you feel unwell, dizzy or light headed top immediately. If you feel ill or pick up an injury then you will need to take a break from the programme to allow your body to recover. If you have concerns about any of the exercises listed in the programme then please do not do them. Ensure you have your doctor's permission before starting this exercise programme.

Programme Schedule

Day	MON	TUES	WED	THURS	FRI	SAT	SUN
	Chest & back	Legs	Shoulders & arms	Rest	Chest & back	Legs	Circuit *

Ensure correct form at all times, full range of motion. If you fail to make the weight increase, go back 1 week and then continue. Good quality reps are more important than sloppy reps.

*Weeks 4, 8 & 11 this becomes an additional rest day

Tempo:
All exercises 3 seconds eccentric and 1 second concentric. So, a set of 10 should take 40 seconds to complete. (This does not apply to the strength circuit exercises).

Warm up suggestion: Use the cross trainer to warm up for 10 minutes start off on with a level of moderate resistance and increase by 1 level each minute. Followed by dynamic stretches and mobility drills.

Warm Up Sets: Prior to starting the work sets, it is recommended that you perform 2-3 warm up sets of a light weight for 12-15 repetitions. Gradually increasing the weight with each set.

Training Protocol: Select a weight that you can complete for the desired number of repetitions without losing form. If you have to cheat to complete the set, then the weight is too heavy. But on the flipside, if the weight is so light that you do not find the last couple of reps challenging, then increase the weight gradually until you do.

Each week, increase the weight by the lowest increment available (usually 1.25kg on each side of the barbell, 2kg for dumbbells.) It is advisable to maintain a training log, so that you know how much weight you are lifting each session and can plan your progression.

For bodyweight exercises such as pull ups and dips, the weight can be increased by adding weight. If the rep range is too high for you to complete those reps then you can use an exercise alternative such as a lat pull down to complete this set.

Note: This is an intermediate / advanced training programme. Trainees should be injury free, have their doctors permission to begin this programme and should have a good foundation of strength and be proficient in the basics such as (but not limited to) squats, deadlifts, bench press, bent over row, pull ups

Chest and Back

Superset	Week 1-4	Weeks 5-8	9-12
Incline Dumbell Press Pull Ups	3 x 10	4 x 8-12	1 x 12 1 x 10 1 x 8 1 x 15
Flat Barbell Bench Press Bent over row	3 x 10	4 x 8-12	1 x 12 1 x 10 1 x 8 1 x 15 (bent over row only) 1 x Strip set (bench press only)
Dips Chin Ups (close grip)	3 x 10	4 x 8-12	1 x 12 1 x 10 1 x 8 1 x 15
Cable Flyes Land Mine Row*	3 x 12 *3 x 8	4 x 15 *4 x 8	2 x 12 2 x 20 *2 x 8 2 x 12
Hanging Leg Raises Cable Pull Down	3 x 12	4 x 15	4 x 20

Legs

Exercise	Week 1-4	Weeks 5-8	9-12
Barbell Back Squat	4 x 10	1 x 12 1 x 10 1 x 8 1 x 15	3 x 8-12 1 x 20
Romanian Deadlift	4 x 10	4 x 8-12	4 x 15
Leg Press	4 x 12	2 x 12 2 x 20	3 x 15 1 x 20
Leg Curl	4 x 12	2 x 12 2 x 15	2 x 15 2 x Failure
Leg Extension	4 x 12	4 x 12	2 x 15 2 x Failure
Calf Raises	4 x 10	4 x 12	4 x 15
Plank	3 x 60 seconds	3 x 90 seconds	3 x 120 seconds

Arms & Shoulders

Exercise	Week 1-4	Weeks 5-8	9-12
Military Press	3 x 10	4 x 10	4 x 10
Lateral cable raises (behind back)	3 x 12	4 x 12	2 x 12 2 x 15
Rear Delt Flyes	3 x 12	4 x 12	2 x 12 2 x 15
Band Pull Aparts	2 x 20	2 x 20	2 x 20
Arm Supersets:			
Standing EZ Bar Curl Tricep Push Down	3 x 10	4 x 12	2 x 8 2 x 12
Isolation Curl Standing Tricep Extension	3 x 10	4 x 12	2 x 12 2 x Forced Reps (eccentric focus)

Strength and Conditioning Circuit

Exercise	Sets / Reps
Dead Lift	3 x 5
Dumbbell Clean & Press	3 x 10
Farmers Walks	4 x 30-50 metres
Tyre Flips	3 x 12 Flips
Prowler / Sled Push	4 x 30-50 metres
Hanging Leg Raises	3 x 12

FAILURE – When you reach the point where you can no longer complete the exercise in the correct manner whilst maintaining proper form. Do not push past the point where form is compromised.

SUPERSET – 2 exercises are performed back-to-back. For example, if bench press is in a superset with bent over row. Perform the bench press and then go and perform the bent over row straight after, that is 1 superset. Take 90-120 seconds rest between each superset.

STRIP SET – Perform the exercise until you cannot complete any more reps without having to cheat) and then quickly strip weight off the bar and perform a set until Failure, strip more weight off the bar and repeat until failure again.

FORCED REPS – Perform the set until failure, then use slight assistance from either your other arm or a training partner for the concentric part of the rep, and then slowly control the eccentric for 3 seconds. Repeat until the assistance is more than what you are able to muster with the muscle that is being trained.

PYRAMID SETS – During the later stages of the programme some exercises will be performed in pyramid fashion. For example:

$$1 \times 12$$
$$1 \times 10$$
$$1x \, 8$$

This means for the working sets the weight should be adjusted based on the rep range. Lighter weights for the higher reps and heavier weights for the lower reps.

Rest days
Go for a walk and do some stretches on your rest days, this will assist your recovery. Aim for 7-8 hours sleep per night, consistently.

Rest Between Sets
90-120 seconds rest between sets

Cardio
20 minutes of cycling at moderate intensity on training days at start of workout, or at another point in the day that is convenient for you.

Progression
You will notice that most workouts progressi in an almost linear fashion, if at any point you cannot keep up with the rate of progression then regress by 1 week and then carry on.

Nutrition
Make sure you are consuming a balanced diet of adequate calories and keeping yourself hydrated.

Protein intake: 1.6 – 1.8g per kg of bodyweight per day
Carbohydrate intake: 4 - 6g per kg of bodyweight per day
Fats: 20 – 30% of daily calorie intake

Post Workout nutrition: A recovery shake with a carbohydrate / protein ratio of 2:1 within 20 mins after training has completed.

Ensure you eat a meal within 1 hour of your training session to ensure the recovery process begins asap.

It is advisable to not drink any alcohol if you wish to make the most amount of progress during this programme.

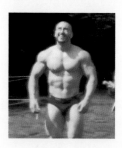

Chest Exercises

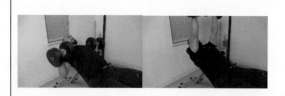	**Incline Dumbbell Press** Press the dumbbells up and slowly lower them down
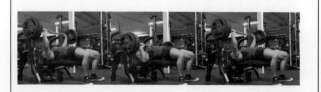	**Barbell Bench Press** Grip bar tight, neutral spine, natural arch on the lower back. Lower the weight down towards the chest and press back up

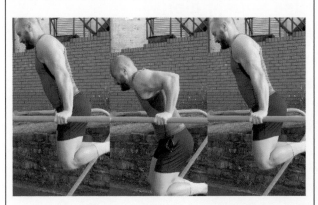

Dips
Using parallel bar, lean forward and slowly lower yourself down as low as your flexibility allows. Upper arm parallel to the floor is fine, then press back up.

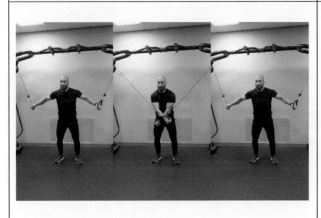

Cable Flyes
Abduct the arms across the chest while holding the cables. Squeeze the pectoral muscles for a second or 2 and then slowly return to the starting position.

Chest Exercise Substitutions

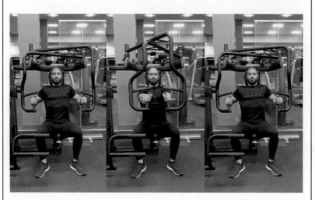	**Chest Press** Ensure your follow specific instructions for the particular machine you are using. Push the hand grips forwards by extending the arms. Squeeze the pectoral muscles and then slowly lower back down.
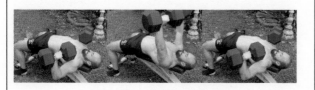	**Dumbbell Bench Press** Keep the arms tucked towards the sides and push upwards by extending the arms and then slowly lower down
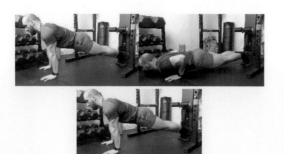	**Press Ups** Hands shoulder width apart elbows tucked in towards the side slowly lower your chest to the floor and then push back up

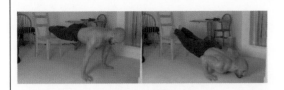	**Incline Press Ups** As above, with feet elevated
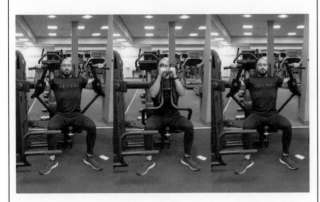	**Pec Deck** Ensure your follow specific instructions for the particular machine you are using. Abduct the arms across the chest while holding the cables. Squeeze the pectoral muscles for a second or 2 and then slowly return to the starting position.

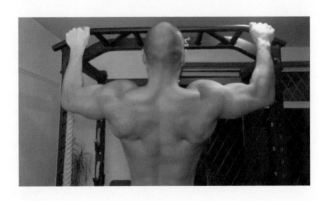

Back Exercises

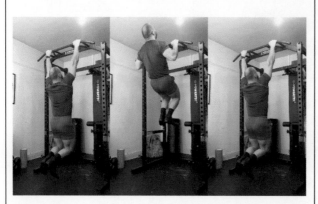

Pull Ups
Grab the bar with an overhand grip with hands slightly wider than shoulder width apart. Hang with your feet off the floor. Pull your chest to the bar and slowly lower down until arms are fully extended.

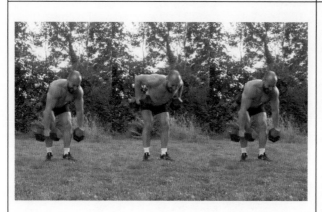

Bent Over Row
(pictured with dumbbells, can be performed with a barbell)
Grip the (barbell) with an overhand grip, drive up using your legs. Stand tall, then push your hips back and bend your knees slightly keeping your chest out.
Row the elbows backwards, bringing the bar towards your stomach. Slowly lower down.

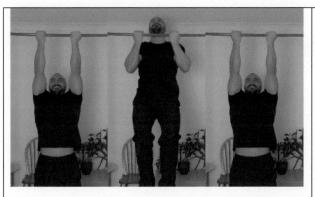

Chin Ups

Grip hold of the bar with palms slightly narrower than shoulder width apart, palms facing towards you.
Pull yourself up until your chin is over the bar and slowly lower yourself down until arms are extended.

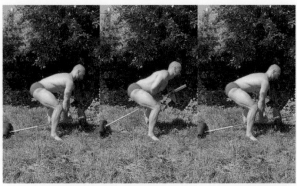

Pictured using a matt weighted down with dumbbells

Landmine Row

Ideally using a landmine attachment. Add the desired weight. Stand with the barbell between your feet, with feet about shoulder width apart or just slightly wider. Push your hips back and bend your knees keeping your spine neutral. Grip the bar (using either a Tbar attachment, V grip, or hand over hand as pictured). Pull your elbows back, pause for a second and slowly lower the weight down and repeat for desired number of repetitions.

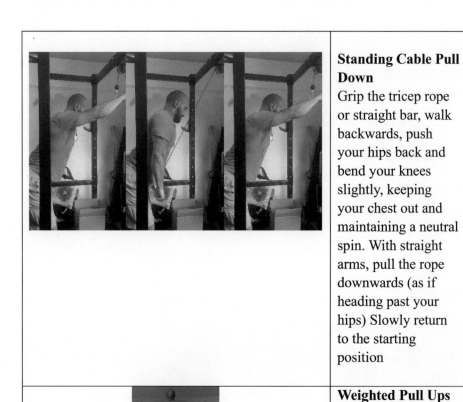	**Standing Cable Pull Down** Grip the tricep rope or straight bar, walk backwards, push your hips back and bend your knees slightly, keeping your chest out and maintaining a neutral spin. With straight arms, pull the rope downwards (as if heading past your hips) Slowly return to the starting position
	Weighted Pull Ups As above pull ups but with either a weighted vest or using a lifting belt.
	Weighted Chin Ups As above chin ups but with either a weighted vest or using a lifting belt.

Back Exercises Substitutions

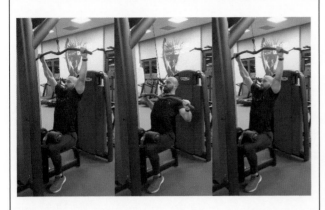

Lat Pull Down
Grip the bar with a wide grip, palms facing towards you. Lean back slightly and stick your chest out. Pull the elbows backwards behind you, bringing the bar to the top of your chest. Slowly control the bar back upwards until the arms are straight and you feel a stretch on the uupper back muscles.

Seated Row Machine
Ensure your follow specific instructions for the particular machine you are using.

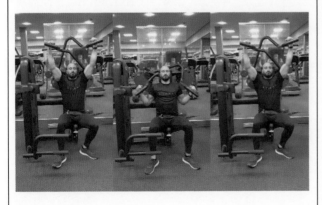

Pull Down Machine
Ensure your follow specific instructions for the particular machine you are using.
Grip the hand grips (neutral grip as pictured here) and pull the elbows down, slowly control up until you feel a stretch on the upper back muscles.

Neutral Grip Pull Ups
Pull up with palms facing towards each other

Leg Exercises

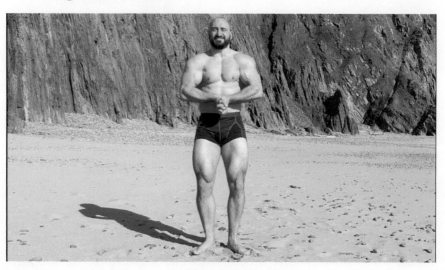

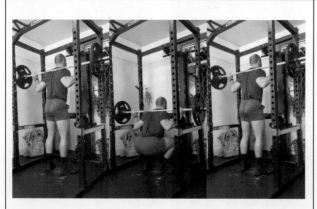

Barbell Back Squat
Feet about shoulder width apart, or (slightly wider) Step backwards from the rack and slowly lower the hips down, keeping your heels on the floor, knees tracking the toes and chest up. Drive back up by extending the legs.

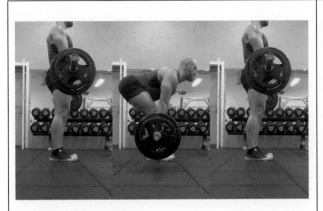

Romanian Deadlift
Grip the bar with an overhand grip, feet about shoulder width apart toes pointing forwards. From the standing position, push your hips back and bend your knees slightly, keeping your chest out. Go until you feel a stretch on the hamstring and then extend back up to the starting position. Keep the bar close to your body.

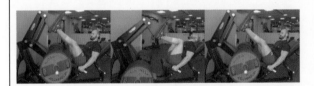

Leg Press
Ensure your follow specific instructions for the particular machine you are using.
Push the plate backwards by extending the legs under control (do not hyperextend the knees) and slowly lower back.

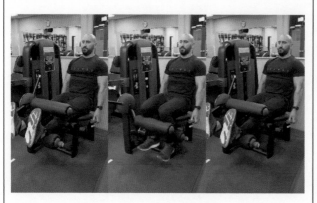	**Leg Curl** Ensure your follow specific instructions for the particular machine you are using. Curl the heel backwards and then slowly straighten the legs until you feel a stretch on the hamstrings.
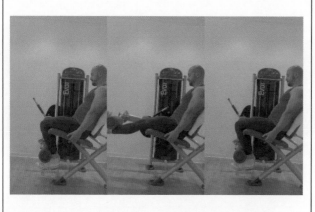	**Leg Extension** Ensure your follow specific instructions for the particular machine you are using. Extend the leg, squeeze the quadriceps and then slowly bend the leg.
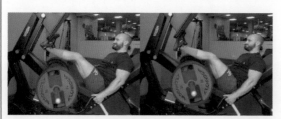 *Pictured using leg press machine*	**Calf Raises** Ensure your follow specific instructions for the particular machine you are using. Slowly lower back until you feel a stretch in the calf and then extend.

Leg Exercises Substitutions

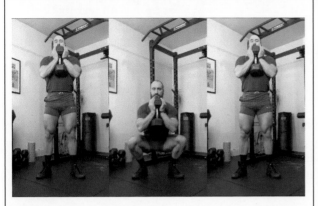

Goblet Squat
Stand tall with feet slightly wider than hip-width distance apart feet slightly turned out.

Look straight ahead and tighten your ab muscles
Bend your knees and sink your hips back while lowering your hips towards the floor. Try to keep a straight spine and tight core throughout the whole movement.
Straighten your legs and drive back up to standing position

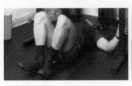 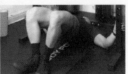

Glute Bridge
Keep neutral spine, shoulder and head flat on the floor. Bring heels back towards your butt and then drive the heels into the floor pushing your hips up and squeezing your glutes at the top of the movement, slowly lower down.

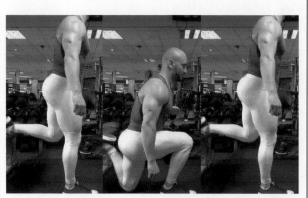

Bulgarian Split Squat
With rear foot elevated, knees tracking the toe, slowly lower yourself down until the kneel is just touching the floor and then drive up with the front leg.

Pictured is a contra-loaded dumbbell

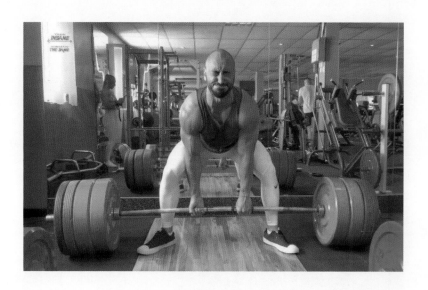

22

Shoulder Exercises

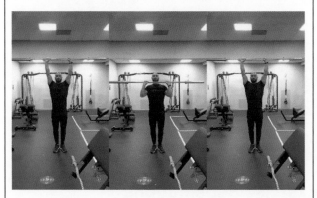	**Military Press** Keep heels together, core tight, squeeze the glutes and quads throughout to provide support and stability. Press the barbell overhead and slowly lower in front of the head until it is just above your shoulders.
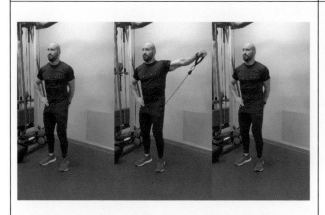	**Lateral Cable Raises** (behind back) Keep your body braced and raise the cable out the side, slow lower down until slightly behind your back
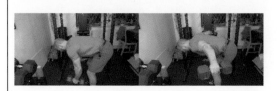	**Rear Delt Flyes** Stand up tall with the dumbbell in each hand to the side. Push your hips back and bend the knees keeping your spine neutral.

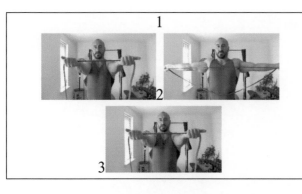	**Band Pull Aparts** Using a light resistance band, palms facing upwards with straight arms out to the front, pull your arms out to the side.

Shoulder Exercise Substitutions

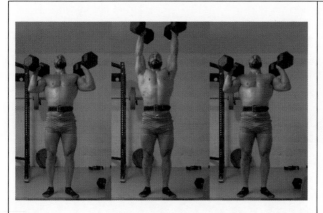	**Dumbbell Press** Keep heels together, core tight, squeeze the glutes and quads throughout to provide support and stability. Grip the dumbbells and extend overhead and slowly lower them back down

Seated Dumbbell Press
As above, but seated on a bench with back supported.

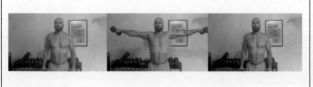	**Lateral Dumbbell Raises** Hold light dumbbells in each hand and slowly raise them to the side with a slight bend in the elbow. Slowly lower them back down.

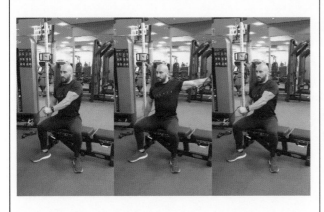

Rear Delt Cable Flyes

Seated on the bench and focussing on one arm at the time, pull the cable towards the side and slowly lower down in front of your body

Arm Exercises

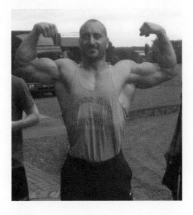

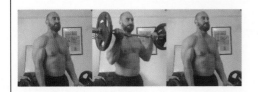

Barbell Curl
Keep your core tight, elbows in towards the side, curl the weight up and then slowly lower down until you feel a stretch on the bicep

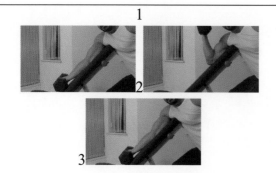 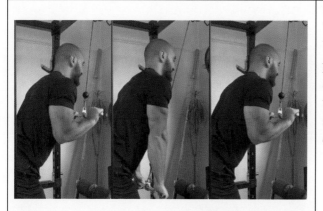	**Isolation Curl** Start off with arm straight, curl the dumbbell upwards and slowly lower down until you feel a stretch on the bicep. The angle of the bench can be adjusted to change the intensity in different parts of the movement.
	Tricep Push Down Upper arm fixed in place, extend the arms, squeeze the tricep and then slowly bend the elbow.
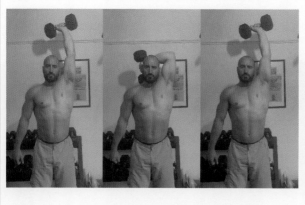	**Standing Over Head Arm Extension** With a single dumbbell, extend it overhead and slowly bend the elbow lower the weight behind your head and then straight out the arm.

Strength Circuit Exercises

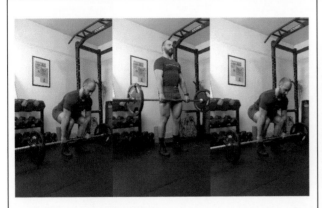

Dead Lift
With feet shoulder width apart toes pointing forwards, grip the bar with an overhand grip Keep your spine straight and drive through your feet extending at the knee and at the hip to stand up keeping the bar close to your body
Push your hips back and bend your knees to lower the bar back down to the floor

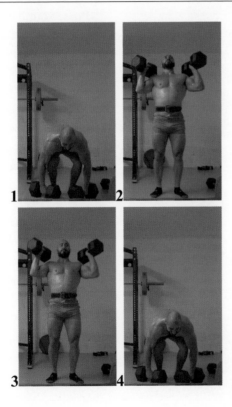

Dumbbell Clean & Press
Position 2 dumbbells on the floor, angled slightly (see picture) (or alternatively start with dumbbell hanging at your sides)
Hinge at the hips and bending at the knees until you can reach the dumbbells. Push your feet into the ground extend your hips and knees and squeeze your glutes and abs. Bringing the weight to shoulder level. Keep core tight, and keep squeezing your glutes, press the weights overhead until the arms are straight. Control the weights down.

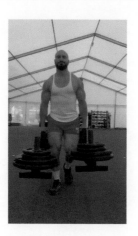	**Farmers Walks** Grip the farmers walk bars in each hand. With feet shoulder width apart and toes pointing forward, dead lift the weight up. Stand tall, chest up, core tight and begin walking forwards, short steps until your reach the desired distance.
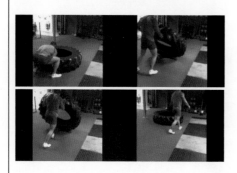	**Tyre Flips** Place your hands under the tyre and with a wide stand, core tight drive up with the legs by pushing the feet into the ground, catch the tyre and then spring into a split stance press it forward to flip it. This is a full body movement.
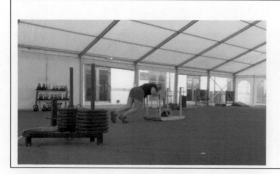	**Prowler / Sled Push** Keep your chest out, neutral spine and drive with the legs

Strength Circuit Exercise Substitutions

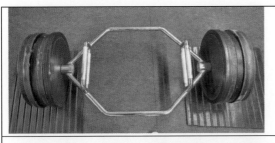

Trap Bar Dead Lift
As deadlift, but using a trap bar, the arms will be by the sides with palms facing inwards.

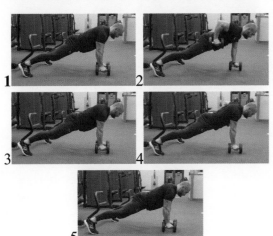

Renegade Row
Adopt the press up position with hands on two dumbbells. With feet slightly wider than shoulder width apart, keep your core tight and control the dumbbell upwards towards your hip by pulling the elbow up, then slowly lower the dumbbell down. Alternate sides, and try and keep your hips and shoulder parallel to the floor thought out. Do not try and rotate or rock side to side to complete the movement, this is an anti-rotation exercise.

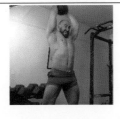

(please note – use a real slam ball, not a medicine ball as the med ball may bounce back in your face)

Slam Ball
Pick the slam ball up and throw it down towards the floor with maximum force.

Sprints
Sprint as fast as you can for the desired distance

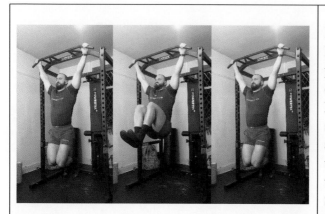

Hanging Leg Raises
Hang from a suitable pull up bar with an overhand grip
Keeping your body stable engage your abs and hip flexors to raise your knees towards your chest
Slowly lower to the starting position
Repeat for desired number of repetitions, and remember this is a controlled movement without swinging

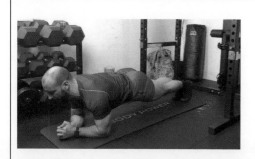

Planks
Elbows below the shoulder
Maintain a straight spine
Keep your core tight and engaged
Focus on your breathing

Passive Stretching

These are stretches assisted by an external force and are typically held for 30 seconds. Passive stretching should be done after the work out.

This guide will display some recommended passive stretches. Gently ease into position and once you feel the stretch hold for 30 seconds and breathe. Do not force the stretch to the point where it becomes painful!

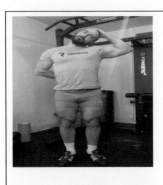	**Trapezius Stretch** 1. Stand upright looking straight ahead 2. Tilt your head to one side 3. Gently apply pressure with your hand until you feel the stretch on the side / rear of your neck 4. Hold for 30 seconds and repeat on the other side
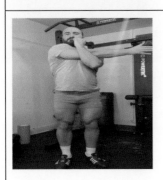	**Shoulder Stretch** 1. Stand upright looking straight ahead 2. Bring your arm across your chest 3. Staying clear of the elbow joint, apply pressure with your other arm until you feel the stretch on your shoulder 4. Hold for 30 seconds and repeat on the other side

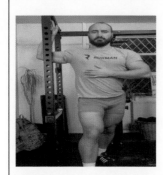	**Chest Stretch** 1. From a standing position place your forearm at an approximate right angle on a wall or squat rack frame 2. Gentle lean your bodyweight forwards until you feel a stretch on the chest 3. Hold for 30 seconds and repeat on the other side
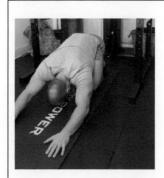	**Back Stretches** 1. On all fours arms straight shoulders directly above the hands and hips above the knees 2. Gently sink your hip down towards your heels and reach your arms out to the front 3. Hold for 30 seconds and then ease out of the stretch to the starting position

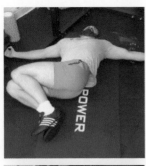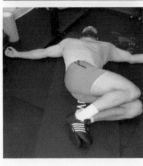	1. Start off lying on your back with head and shoulder on the floor 2. Bend the knees and slowly turn your pelvis to one side, keeping feet and knees together 3. Go until you feel the stretch and hold for 30 seconds and then repeat on the other side
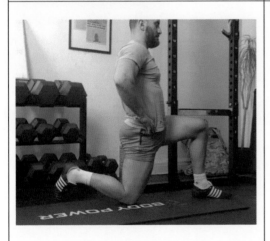	**Hip Flexor Stretch** 1. Place your right knee on the floor and your left foot out to the front, slightly forward of the left knee 2. Tense your right glute as hard as you can throughout stretch 3. Slowly bring your hips forwards until your feel a stretch on the top of your right thigh 4. Hold for 30 seconds, ease backwards out of the stretch and repeat on the other side

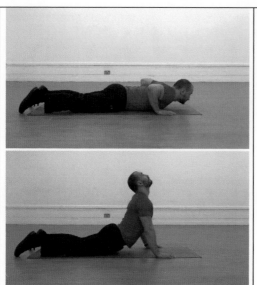	**Abdominal and Hip Flexor Stretch** 1. Lie on your front, hands directly below the shoulders 2. Tense your glutes as hard as you can throughout the entire stretch 3. Slowly extend your arms as far as you comfortably can 4. Hold for 15-30 seconds 5. Slowly lower back down
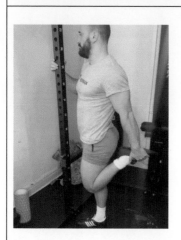	**Quadricep Stetch** 1. From either a standing or lying position 2. Bend at the knee and take charge of your foot with you hand pulling your heel towards your glute 3. Keep knees in line and push the hips forward until you feel a stretch on the front of the thigh 4. Hold for 30 seconds and repeat on the other side

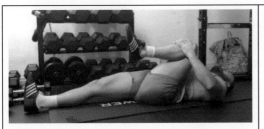	**Hamstring – Glute Stretch Routine** 1. Lie on your back with both legs straight 2. Bring your left knee up towards your torso 3. Apply press on your shin to increase stretch 4. Hold for 30 seconds
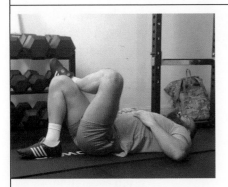	1. Release the above stretch 2. Bend your right knee and place foot flat on the floor 3. Bring your left foot inwards so the side of the left shin is rested on the right thigh just below the knee 4. Hold for 30 seconds to stretch the glute. 5. To increase the stretch follow the below protocol, or; 6. Release the stretch and repeat this and the previous stretch on the opposite side

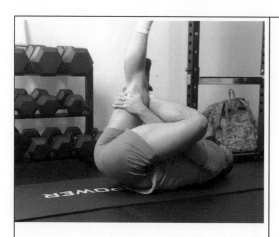	1. From the above position 2. Place both hands on your right hamstring just below the knee and straighten your right leg pointing upwards towards the ceiling 3. Gently lean backwards until you feel an increased stretch on the left glute 4. Hold for 30 seconds and repeat the 3 stretches on the other side
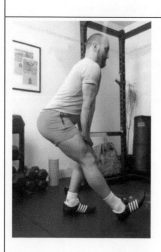	**Hamstring Stretch** 1. From a standing position 2. Step your right foot forwards keeping your right leg straight 3. Maintain a neutral spine, place your hands on the left thigh above the knee 4. Slowly sit back bending your leg knee and lowering your hips until your feel a stretch on the straight right leg 5. Hold for 30 seconds and repeat on the other side

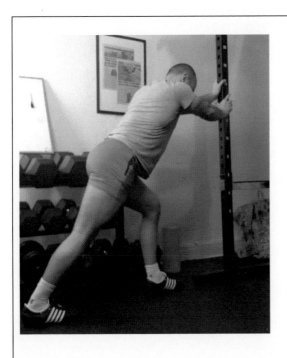

Calf Stretch

1. Face a wall or solid framed object such a squat rack
2. Place both hands on the wall (or frame as pictured)
3. With a staggered stance and both toes pointing forwards and heels on the floor
4. Slowly start to shift your hips forwards whilst firmly keeping your rear heel on the floor until your feel a stretch on your rear calf
5. Hold for 30 seconds, gently ease out of the stretch and repeat on the other side

If you are unsure of the correct technique on how to perform any of these exercises check with a qualified trainer in your gym to check that you are doing the exercises correctly.

Basic Nutrition Information

I have included, as a guide a typical daily meal plan that I would use when doing this training programme. This is by no means a perfect diet plan, however I try and maintain a very simple approach to nutrition.

My basis for planning meals will typically involve:

- A protein element
- A carbohydrate element
- A fat element
- A "healthy" element

Protein

Protein is composed of amino acids, and is the building blocks of muscle mass. Foods that are protein rich include:

- Dairy products such as eggs, milk, cottage cheese
- Meat
- Poultry
- Seafood
- Beans
- Seeds, nuts

A healthy and safe amount of protein ranges from 0.8 – 2 grams of protein per kilogram of bodyweight. Extremely active athletes may require the upper end of this spectrum however most normal people will not need so much.

Carbohydrates

Carbs are the body's primary energy source. Good quality

carbohydrates can fuel your training and increase performance.

- Whole grains such as oats, bread
- Sweet potatoes
- Yams
- Brown rice
- Wholewheat pasta

Fruits such as bananas and berries are good sources of quick carbohydrates, that could be used as pre or post workout, however for your main meals try and stick to the complex carbs.

Picking nutrient dense food such as beetroot to your plate can be really useful.

Fats

While typically avoided, fat is an essential part of a healthy and balanced diet. It is a source of essential fatty acids and plays an important role in the absorption of many vitamins.

The main type of fats are:
- Saturated fats
- Unsaturated fats

It is recommended that we try and consume less saturated fats by replacing them with unsaturated fats within our daily fat intake.

- Avocados
- Nuts and seeds
- Oily fish such as sardines, mackerel, salmon, trout

"Healthy" Element

I would always aim to try and have some kind of fruit or vegetables on my plate to assist with vitamin and mineral intake. This could include:

- Vegetables such as broccoli, carrots, cauliflower, peas, sweetcorn, beetroot
- Fruit such as bananas, apples, grapefruit, watermelon, oranges
- Salad

Note: the "healthy" element could fall into one of the other categories listed such as avocados would also fall into the fat category, or beetroot could be used as the carbohydrate element.

Supplements

Caffeine – Can offer a pre-workout boost (no need to take any fancy powders, a cup of coffee should suffice)

Creatine – Can allow some people to perform better at high intensity sessions such as weight lifting. Optimum dosage would be at 5g per day post workout.

Whey protein – to assist with muscle repair following intense training sessions

Magnesium – Assists with nerve function, energy and muscle contractions. Optimum time to take this very important mineral as a supplement would be before bed as it can help you relax and sleep better, assisting with enhanced recovery.

Supplements cannot replace a complete, healthy balanced diet. So before even considering taking any supplements make sure that you have your nutrition in check.

Sample Meal Plan

This is how I would prepare my meals. For periods where I want to put on weight, I would increase the carbohydrate element. To cut down on weight I would gradually decrease my carbohydrate element.

Meal 1
1 apple
6 scrambled eggs (with milk)
Porridge oats (with water, pumpkin seeds, sunflower seeds and blueberries)
Glass of orange juice
1 banana

Meal 2
1 banana
2 x Chicken breast
Sweet potato
Mixed veg – broccoli, carrots, sweet corn
Glass of whole milk

Meal 3
1 satsuma
Fish (either salmon, tuna, sardines)
Pasta
Mixed vegetables / salad
Glass of whole milk

Meal 4
Beef steak / burger (5% fat)
Quinoa
Salad – lettuce, carrots (no sauce)
1 Avocado

Meal 5
300g cottage cheese
2 kiwi fruits
Cup of warm milk (before bed)

This meal plan would not be the exact same each day, but would be similar. So, for example some days I may change the specific food around but the elements would remain the same, so for example some days I may have an additional chicken breast instead of the beef in meal 4. Or rice instead of pasta.

After training I would have 1 banana and a pint of milk. Whey protein supplement could be used in replacement of milk.

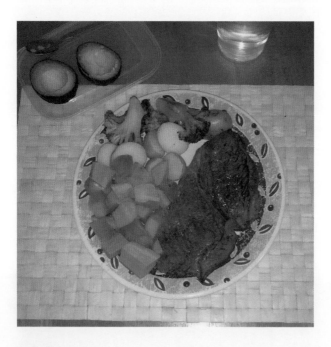

Meal Prep

Meal prep is absolutely essential if you want to ensure you stick to your nutrition plan. Spending an hour or so a week to prepare as many meals as you can for the week ahead can play huge dividends, especially if you are busy.

I found it best to make a huge batch of different meals, putting them into little containers and putting my meals for the next two days in the fridge and for days 3-6 I'd put them in the freezer, bringing them out 24 hours before and moving them to the fridge.

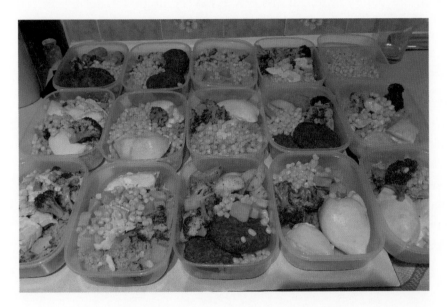

These days I try and opt for glass containers rather than plastic ones. Storing and cooking food in plastic containers can leech chemicals into your food which you then consumer and this can have knock on effects on the endocrine system.

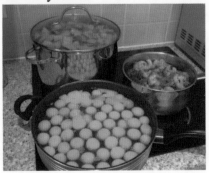

Rest

Why is rest important? When you train your body responds in the period of time after training to adapt and get fitter. If you trained hard every single day, partied every night surviving on less than 2 hours sleep only to repeat this process every single day for a year what sort of state do you think you would be in?

Rest falls into a few categories:

Rest During a Workout

This is the period where you take breaks during your exercise. The harder and more intense the exercise is the more rest period you would likely require. For example, a powerlifter who is lifting nearly 100% of their 1 rep max would require more rest than someone who was lifting 50% of their 1 rep max. (1 RM= the most you can lift in one go).
As you get fitter, the less rest period you will require. Someone who is unfit, new to training or recovering from an injury will require a longer rest period.

Rest Days (and when not exercising)

Rest days (or the remainder of the training day) does not mean lying in bed all day doing nothing. Ideally try and limit the amount of stress you put on your body. You will likely not be able to recover as quickly from an intense training session if you're also spending another few hours playing sports or some other intense activity. However, performing light forms of exercise such as walking or stretching will be beneficial and could assist recovery and improve your physical and mental wellbeing. I am not saying do not participate in any sports, however I would suggest adjusting your programme to accommodate for the sport in such a way that neither your running training or your extra-curricular activity does not suffer as a consequence.

A lot of this does come down to prioritising your goals. Many of us would love to be able to participate in several sports at a high level, build muscle, lose bodyfat, lift the big boy weights, run marathons and sprint the 100m like Usain Bolt. However, we simply cannot be as master of all trades. Especially when we consider things like work, family, children, hobbies and other commitments we may have.

According the SAID principle, the human body adapts specifically to imposed demands.

Specific
Adaption to
Imposed
Demands

This means that to get the best out of your training, it should be focussed around that specific goal. If you are training for several different things at the same time, your body is not able to excel at each one, as it doesn't know what it needs to adapt to!

Sleep

Sleep is a very important function of the body. It allows the brain and body to recharge, keeps the body and mind healthy and functioning correctly. Regular poor sleep can increase your chances of obesity, heart disease and diabetes. Health experts also warn that it can shorten your life expectance. This shows that sleep is absolutely fundamental in allowing our bodies to function and perform at an optimum level. Consistent lack of sleep can lower your testosterone levels, reduce your immune system and obliterate your sex drive. If you have ever been a shift worker or served in the military you will know a thing or two about sleep deprivation. However, many individuals from these backgrounds believe they do not need to sleep 8 hours per night to function. They state that they are used to it, and well… they are part right.

The human body is absolutely amazing at adapting to whatever is thrown at it. So, in the case of the shift worker who operates on a handful of hours sleep here and there, they are actually in a perpetual state of tiredness. The only thing is – their bodies have got used to feeling tired and so feeling tired becomes normal.

Can you remember a time 2 years ago and remember how tired or awake you were feeling on a given day and compare it with how tired you are today? Unlikely. Can you compare how tired or awake you felt yesterday and compare it with how tired today? Quite possibly.

An individual who consistently gets less than 6 hours sleep can suffer the same drop in performance over a period of 2 weeks as an individual who sleeps 8 hours a week suffers by staying awake for over 24 hours. The difference is the person getting 8 hours sleep notices it – feels like trash, whereas the person who is consistently sleep deprived does not notice it due to the gradual decline and the "renorming" process.

So yes, we can get used to not sleeping, however the health consequences will be building up underneath the surface.

If you need further convincing what this also means is if you don't get enough quality sleep:
1. Your running will not improve to its full potential
2. Your testosterone will dramatically decrease – even if you are young and healthy (it's worse for anyone over 30 too!)
3. You're more likely to get injured and be sick

Beyond Hercules Programme

You have completed the 12 week programme… well done! This section is here to help you build upon the progress you have made and empower you to design your own training programme.

Here's what you need to do:

1. Establish what your goal is, write this down
2. Determine how many days you are able to train per week
3. Ideally, you should be able to train a body part at 2-3 times per week. Your programme will need to reflect this so you will have to come up with a "split" that is suitable
4. Select exercises that are specific to your needs. For example you want to build bigger rear delts on the shoulders then you would need exercises that specifically target that area such as rear delt flyes
5. Progress the exercise by gradually increasing the weight. After about 4 weeks, change things up. This can be done by either adjusting the exercise slightly, increasing the volume, changing the rep range or performing advanced techniques such as pyramid sets, super sets, rest/pause sets etc.

Rest / Pause set

The rest / pause set is an intensity technique that can be used to challenge the muscles and force them to grow bigger and stronger. It is advisable not to do this on exercises like the squat or deadlift as it requires you to go to failure a few times during the one set. For other exercises such as bench press it would be a good idea to have a spotter with you, just in case.

As always, ensure you have warmed up adequately before you begin your working set.

- Set a weight of 80-85% of your 1 rep max

- Perform as many reps as possible until you reach failure
- Rest for 3 breaths
- Perform as many reps as possible until you reach failure
- Rest for 3 breaths
- Perform as many reps as possible until you reach failure

For example

<u>Set 1</u> 8 reps
<u>Set 2</u> 3 reps
<u>Set 3</u> 2 reps

Total:13 reps

Training Splits

Here are some typical bodybuilding splits

- Full body routine
- 2 day split
- 5 day split
- Push, Pull, Legs

<u>Full Body Routine</u>

This is an ideal routine for a beginner and is performed three times per week. The focus should be on compound exercises that target the whole body for example:

- Squats
- Romanian deadlift

- Bench press
- Pull Ups
- Bent over row
- Shoulder press

Each exercise should be performed for 3 working sets, gradually increasing the weight each week. Full body routines are an excellent way of building muscle and a foundation of strength.

2 Day Split

A typical 2 day split routine would be performed ideally four times a week:

- Workout 1 – Upper body
- Workout 2 – Lower body

Each workout should start with compound exercises and the same principle of progressive overload applied. Then 1 or 2 isolation exercises can be selected at the end of the workout and performed for a higher rep range of 12-15 repetitions.

5 Day Split

This is more of an advanced bodybuilding workout routine, that involves high volume for each body part on that specific day. The target muscle group if blasted for that session with more exercises than would be in the previous 2 splits. For example:

- **Day 1:** Legs
- **Day 2:** Chest
- **Day 3:** Back
- **Day 4:** Rest
- **Day 5:** Shoulders
- **Day 6:** Arms
- **Day 7:** Rest

Leg day is put first when the body is fresh as this should be the hardest session. Abs would typically be trained with a couple of exercises as the end of each session.

Select 4-5 exercises per body part.

When designing a 5 day split it is important to note that muscles do work together and that muscles other than the "target" muscle group will be worked. For example on Back day – the biceps and forearms will be worked. This is why arms are on day 6, so that they should be recovered by the time chest and back days arrive. It would not make sense to put arms day the day before chest or back as this could compromise your main compound lifts for those respective days and result in your target muscle group for that day not being trained effectively.